The day Aunt Flo Comes to Visit

An Honest Conversation About Getting Your Period

by

Dr. Janell L. Carroll

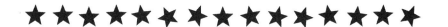

International Standard Book Number ISBN-13: 978-0-9798549-0-3,
ISBN-10: 0-9798549-0-3

Design and Layout
MAS Designs
PO Box 156
Avon, Connecticut 06001

To my daughters,
Reagan and MacKenzie,
with the wish that girls in their
generation will be free to embrace
all aspects of being a girl.

Thank You!

A book like this could never be written without the help
of many talented and supportive family members and
friends. My husband now knows more about periods than
he ever thought he wanted to know. Reagan and Kenzie
offered lots of advice along the way and made sure I knew
when I didn't sound "cool."

A big thank you to Maryann Sheehan for her design and
ideas. Her ability to view the world in a creative light always
leaves me in awe. Another creative soul, Meghan S. Waskowitz,
was an integral piece in making Aunt Flo a reality. There were
many others who helped – big hugs to Lisa & Ariel Lepito,
Lisa Belval, Jeff Roy, Kate & Megan Schuppe, Lynne & Andrea
Swanson, Lauren Bayersdorfer, and Dr. Julie Malkin.

ConTents

★ ★ ★ ★ ★ ★ ★ ★ ★ ★ ★

Note from the Author

My name is Dr. Janell Carroll and I wrote this book for girls just like you - girls who are growing up and becoming women. Although you're probably really excited about all these changes, you might also be feeling kind of confused and maybe even a little scared. Change, although exciting, isn't necessarily easy. It can be scary to walk over a long bridge without knowing exactly what's on the other side. That's what puberty is like. You begin these changes without knowing what will happen and what your body will look and feel like when you get to the other side. Will you get taller? Bigger? Thinner? Stronger? Some girls are thrilled to have these changes happening in their bodies while others wish they could wait a little longer for it all to begin. Either way, knowing what to expect makes things easier.

When I was your age, I had a lot of questions about my first period. I wondered when it would come and how it would feel. I wondered where I would be when it came and I worried....would I be in the middle of Spanish class? Would I be wearing white pants? Would everyone know? The truth is that I had lots of questions (and worries) about my first period!

Worrying about your period is very normal and I'm sure that you have your share of questions, just like I did. Your experiences with your first period will be shaped by how well-informed you are about menstruation. This makes it really important to learn as much as you can. I hope that you've already talked to your mom, dad, grandma, sister, friend, or a relative about what to expect when you get your first period. Maybe you've even had a class in your school that explains menstruation.

This book will really help you understand your period. First we'll look at common questions that girls have about their periods. Then we'll explore the why, what, when, and hows associated with them. Finally, we'll hear from some girls who have had a first period and we'll learn what their experience was like. You'll learn what they thought about, worried about, and where they were when their first period came. Some of these girls had positive experiences and some had negative ones. Some felt excited and some felt scared. The common thread in all of their stories is a wish that they would have been more prepared and knew more about what to expect. In fact, that is what inspired me to write this book. I want you to have more information so that you'll feel more comfortable and confident about the changes that will go on in your body.

My approach throughout this book will be very straightforward. I want you to imagine we're having a conversation together. I will answer your questions with honesty and tell you everything you need to know. I'll even throw in a bit of humor to make you smile every once in awhile!

One more thing.....you might wonder how I came up with the title of this book. When I was young, my friends and I were really embarrassed by menstruation. We didn't want people to hear us talking about our periods. So we came up with a "code" word to talk about it without others knowing what we were talking about. When we had our period we would say "Aunt Flo came to visit." When my best friend Kathy sat down at the lunch table and announced, "Aunt Flo came this morning and she was in a bad mood," we knew that Kathy's Aunt was nowhere to be found. Kathy got her period and was having some bad cramps. Girls still use "code" words like this today and we'll talk about some of these words.

I hope you enjoy reading this book as much as I've enjoyed writing it. If you have any comments or questions, feel free to contact me through my website below. Remember, getting your period is a big event. It is definitely something to be celebrated (…think cake, ice cream, and a big party!)

Warmly,

Dr. Janell Carroll
www.drjanellcarroll.com

Chapter 1

The Basic Questions:
First Periods and What to Do

I have talked with hundreds of girls about their first period. I've talked to young girls who haven't had it yet, girls who just got it, and girls who have had it for years. Throughout these many conversations, I learned that girls have lots of basic questions about their first period. They want to know when it will come, what it will feel like, and how long it will last. I've pulled together the most common questions that girls have asked, and answered them in this chapter. I am sure you'll find that you've asked some of these questions yourself!

when? WHY? does it hurt? tampon or pad?

When will my period come?

It's impossible to pin-point when **menstruation** will begin. One of the best things to do is to ask your mom* when her first period came. The age at which your mom got her period will probably be similar to the age at which you start yours. But maybe your mom doesn't remember or maybe you don't feel comfortable asking her.

Most girls start their periods around the age of 12-13 years old, but some get it earlier and some get it later. Getting your period is often dependent upon your weight, so it may be that you have a little growing left to do. The bottom line is that periods come when our bodies are ready for them. Because of this, there is no right or wrong age to start your period!

REMINDER!!
Important terms are highlighted throughout this book. Look for a glossary of terms (with pronunciations) at the end.

*Throughout this book I will refer to your "mom" and "dad" as your primary caregivers. However, I know that some of you are parented by a single father or a stepparent, parental partner, grandparent, or other extended family member. When I say "mom" and "dad," I am referring to those people who take the responsibility for your care and upbringing.

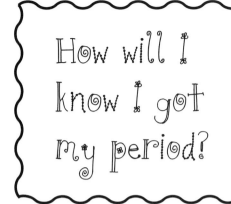

How will I know I got my period?

When you get your first period you'll probably notice a dark colored stain on your underwear. It won't be bright red, even though it has some blood in it. Typically it's a brownish-red color (some girls describe it as rust-colored). You might also see it when you wipe yourself after you go to the bathroom.

If you ignore the stain in your underwear, you'll probably notice another stain the next day. This is typical in a first period because there usually isn't any significant **menstrual flow** until you've had your period a couple of times.

How do I tell my mom that I got my period?

Most girls do tell their mom when they get their period. In fact, I've found that over 87% of girls share the good news with their moms. However, not all moms respond in the same way - some don't make a big deal of it while others are so excited they can hardly contain themselves. Your mom's reaction probably comes from her own experience with her mom.

Some girls are embarrassed to tell their moms they got their period. This is especially true when there hasn't been much communication about puberty and growing up. It can be difficult to talk about these issues. However, it's important to keep in mind that once upon a time your mom was waiting for her first period to come – just like you.

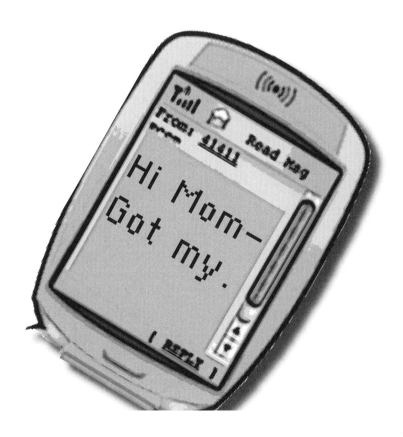

I definitely think you should tell your mom (and your dad too, but we'll talk more about him in a minute). Try telling your mom when she's alone – maybe catch her while she's in her bedroom, bathroom, or while the two of you are driving somewhere. It might help to start the conversation by asking her how old she was when she got her period. In this conversation you can tell her you've started yours. Most moms feel both happy and sad when their daughter gets her first period – it's a big day for them too!

Daddy's
~~Little~~ BIG!!
Girl

But what about telling dad? I really think you should tell him too. I know you probably think he wouldn't care, but you might be surprised. Many dads today want to be more involved and would be really touched that their daughter shared the news with them. In my talks with girls, about 20% of girls told their dad when they got their first period. Their dads were happy and excited to hear the news and were genuinely interested in their daughters' experiences. If you don't feel comfortable talking to your dad about the arrival of your first period, you can ask your mom or another adult to share the news with him.

What will my first period feel like?

You probably won't even notice any symptoms of your first period until you see the stain in your under-wear or on the toilet paper. Most girls do not have any emotional or physical symptoms that alert them that their period is coming. For those who do, they say they felt slight **cramps** or a little more moody or sensitive than usual before their period. Again, everyone is different! As you get older you'll probably experience more physical symptoms with your period and you'll get better at rec-ognizing the symptoms just before your period comes each month.

FastFact
First periods often come without any warning.

Girls who have had their periods for a couple of years usually can tell when a period is going to come. They might notice back cramps or stiffness, breast soreness or fullness, an increase in headaches, bloating, or changes in their sleep patterns. Not all girls experience these symptoms and it's important to pay attention to your own body to figure out how your body lets you know about an upcoming period.

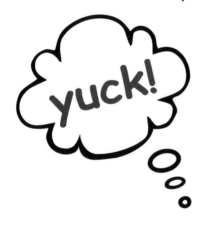

How much blood will be in my underwear the first time?

Menstrual flow is usually fairly sparse during your first period. In fact, you might just see a stain or spotting in your underwear for the first few periods. A common fear that many girls have is that the blood will be flowing heavily and they won't have time to get to the bathroom. This won't happen - you will have plenty of time to get to a bathroom when you get your period the first time.

As you get older, your menstrual flow will increase. Older girls who have had their period for a couple of months lose about 3-5 tablespoons of menstrual fluids during an average period. The fluid can be bright red or dark brown, with a smooth or thick texture. All of this is normal.

What should I do if I start my period in school?

The best thing to do would be to excuse yourself and go the bathroom. Stop by your locker and get a pad if you have one. If not, in the bathroom, take about 5-6 sheets of toilet paper, stack them on top of each other and put them in your underwear. This way the toilet paper can absorb the fluid in your underwear and any additional menstrual fluids that are released. If you are nervous, have cramps, or don't feel well, ask your teacher if you can visit the school nurse.

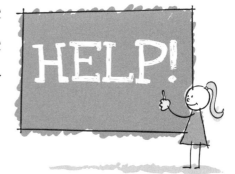

What should I do if I start my period at night?

Don't worry! The menstrual flow probably won't be heavy so you can just get out of bed and either put a pad in your underwear or get some toilet paper. You'll probably want to tell your mom, so decide if you want to wake her at night or wait until morning. If you did get some blood on your sheets you can just wait until morning, rinse them in cool water, and put them in the washer.

Will anyone know that I started my period?

There is absolutely no way for someone to know that you have your period unless you tell them. There are no secret vibes that you give off or special ways someone might "know" without you telling them.

How long will my first period last?

Your first period may only last a day or so. The next couple of periods may not last long either. Some girls have short periods that only last a day or two, while others have longer periods that last a few days. Typically, the first few days of your menstrual cycle are the heaviest flow days and there might only be light spotting for the rest of the cycle. As you get older and your periods become more established, they may last four or five days.

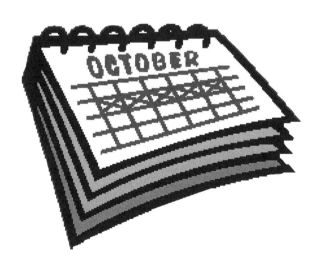

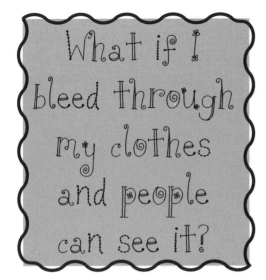

What if I bleed through my clothes and people can see it?

Believe me, every woman I know has this fear! It's very common to worry about this, but you can be prepared. Some girls make sure to keep a sweatshirt in their locker and they tie it around their waist when they have their period. Or they wear dark clothing during the week when their period is due. Making sure that you mark your calendar and chart your cycles can help reduce the likelihood of this happening. If it does, however, just excuse yourself to the bathroom or the nurse's office. Try to be as confident as you can and remember that most of us who have experienced such embarrassment laugh about it one day!

Is it possible to lose too much blood during a period?

Some girls lose more blood than others. Typically, a girl loses anywhere from a few spoonfuls to about a ¼ cup of fluid in a period. Girls who do bleed a lot during a period might be at risk for an iron deficiency and may need to talk to a doctor or medical provider to see if they need iron supplements.

Is it true that you could be too skinny to get your period?

Yes! If a girl drops below a certain weight she might not get her first period. This is common in girls who are serious gymnasts or long-distance runners. Your body has to have a certain level of body fat in order to have a healthy menstrual cycle.

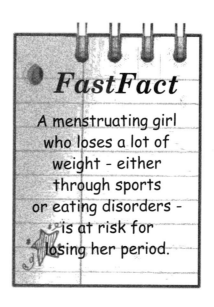

FastFact

A menstruating girl who loses a lot of weight - either through sports or eating disorders - is at risk for losing her period.

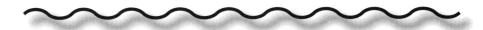

Now you know the basics. Periods really shouldn't be surrounded in mystery and secrecy. They are a very normal part of growing up and there is nothing to be nervous or worried about. In fact, you should feel GREAT that you are a woman. You are a wonderfully unique person and your body is preparing to make you even more terrific. But there is much more to learn! In the next chapter we'll talk about more specifics, such as what to do when you take a bath or go swimming.

Chapter 2

The Special Questions:

Bathing, Swimming, Pads and Tampons

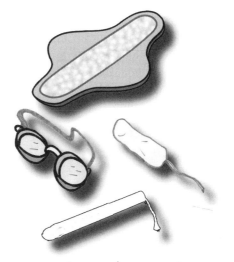

Now that you've got the basics down, it's time to talk about specifics. Here we'll talk about questions such as how often your period will come, whether you can take a bath or go swimming, and how to use pads and tampons. If you think of additional questions while you're reading please ask your mom or another trusted adult. It's very natural to have questions and you deserve answers!

Now that I've had my first period, how often will my period come?

The word "menstruation" comes from the Latin word menses, which means "month." This is because once your periods are regular they come about once a month. That's why some girls say *"it's that time of the month"* when they are having a period. The menstrual cycle is often based on a 28-day cycle which is counted from the first day you start bleeding until the first day of your next period (for example, if you got your period on January 6th and then again on January 31st, your cycle would be 25 days long)

Having a cycle that is more or less than the typical 28-day cycle is perfectly normal. Some girls have 24-day cycles, while others have 30 or 35-day cycles.

1 2 3 4 5 6 7 8 9 10 11 12 13 14 15 16 17

When you first start having a period, your cycles will be fairly irregular. It might be impossible to calculate when a period will come because it may be early one month and then late the next. You might even skip a cycle. All of this is very normal.

As you develop and grow, your cycles will become more regular. When you get older you will usually be able to predict your cycles and know when to expect your period. It's a good idea to mark down your period start and end dates in a calendar. You can also mark down whether the flow is light, medium, or heavy. Once you've kept track for a couple of months, you will have an idea of how many days are between each period and when to expect them. I've included a calendar at the end of this book so you can begin charting your period.

18 19 20 21 22 23 24 25 26 27 28 29 30

Irregular cycles can be caused by several things, including prescription medicines, excessive exercise, low body weight, or dieting. Although much less common, irregular periods can also be due to hormonal imbalances. If you experience irregular cycles for more than two years, you should see a doctor to check hormone levels and make recommendations to help you establish regular periods.

Will I still be able to go to gym when I have my period?

Many girls think that when they have their period they can't participate in gym or activities such as soccer, biking, or running. This just isn't true! Period days are just like any other days, so you can do whatever activities you feel up for. The American College of Obstetrics and Gynecology (a fancy group that does lots of research on periods) has found no reason for menstruation to interfere with a woman's daily activities, including exercise. Having your period is a normal part of your life, so don't let it interfere with your enjoyment of other activities....we'll talk about this next!.

Can you take a bath when you are menstruating? What about swimming in the ocean?

Great questions! Yes, you can bathe, shower, and swim when you have your period. While you don't need to wear a tampon in the shower, you might want to use one if you take a bath or go swimming. This might depend on where you are in your cycle, since your heaviest days of menstrual flow will be the first day or two. Using a tampon when you swim is a safe way to avoid possible leakage. In fact, during normal menstrual flow, a tampon can absorb for over four hours. If it's a heavy flow day just make sure you change the tampon every hour or so. Don't worry about the tampon absorbing the pool water – it is too deep inside the vagina to be able to absorb any water.

Some girls get so worried about their period that they stop swimming. I swam on a swim team for many years and I remember having friends quit when they got their periods. They worried about blood leaking into the pool and their anxieties got the better of them. There is absolutely no reason you cannot swim during your period. You will just need to learn how to use tampons (we'll talk more about this later). Do not be afraid!

I've also talked to girls who told me they stopped swimming in the ocean during their periods because of sharks. While we do know that sharks are attracted to bodily fluids, including blood, we also know that lots of women safely swim in the ocean during their menstrual periods (that reminds me about the old wive's tale about bears.....you don't have to worry about camping while you have your period either. Bears are not attracted to a girl with her period!) Bleeding during menstruation is minimal and occurs over several days, so you're safe around sharks and bears (well, at least as safe as you can be if you're hanging out with wild animals!)

Should I use pads or tampons?

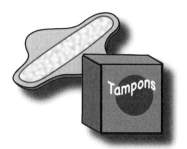

Once you start menstruating, you'll need to use something to absorb the menstrual flow – either a pad or a tampon. Some girls use only pads, some only tampons, and some use both. Sometimes girls use tampons during the day and pads at night. Girls who are really active and involved in sports often like to use tampons during their sporting events and practices.

During your first couple of periods it's probably better to use only pads. That way you'll learn what your typical flow is like. After a couple of months you can decide what you want to use. The decision about what to use is up to you and it's a good idea to talk to your mom or other trusted adults for advice. Tampons can be used at any age but younger girls often have a smaller vaginal opening, making tampons more difficult to use. In order to use tampons, you must be comfortable touching the vaginal area to insert and remove them, and you must be responsible enough to remember to change them frequently. If you are uncomfortable touching your vagina or you are forgetful, tampons might not be for you.

What happens if a pad falls out of my underwear while I'm walking somewhere?

Let's talk first about how to use a pad. Today's pads come with a sticky adhesive on one side covered with a protective strip (you're really lucky because the pads my mom first gave me didn't have sticky stuff - you had to use a crazy belt around your waist to keep the pad in your underwear. Ask your mom if she remembers the old belted pads!!)

When you're ready to use a pad just pull off the protective strip that covers the adhesive and firmly apply it to the inside of your underwear. The sticky adhesive should hold it in place. There are tons of different types of pads available – it's best to try a variety and see what you like best. Some fancy pads come with "wings" so you can fold the sticky stuff around the center of your underwear to prevent staining.

Make sure your underwear fit you properly when using a pad. If you have loose or baggy underwear and you're moving around a lot, the pad could work its way free. Most pads have enough sticky stuff to keep them sticky (unless, of course, you've got a lot of baby powder in your underwear.....this can make it impossible for the pad to stick). If you are in a situation in which your pad does work its way free, the best thing to do is quickly pick up the pad and put it in the trash. If you don't make a big deal of it, no one else will either.

One girl I talked to had a pad fall out of her underwear as she was walking to the front of her class. She calmly turned around, walked back to the runaway pad, stepped on it (it was sticky-side up) and shuffled out of the room with it stuck to her shoe. She was so calm and cool about it, no one really knew what happened!

How do you use a **tampon?**

Tampons are made of absorbent cotton and are inserted in the vagina to absorb menstrual flow. There are many different kinds of tampons - some are designed for light, medium, and heavy flow days and they may be scented or unscented. Some tampons have applicators, which can help you to insert them in the vagina, and some don't. When you first start using tampons it's a good idea to start with the smallest tampons available and use an applicator.

1. Before you insert a tampon, always wash your hands and make sure you won't be interrupted by a nosy brother or sister. You'll want to take your time and not feel rushed or nervous that someone might knock or try to come in the room.

DO NOT DISTURB

A standing position usually works best to insert the tampon and you might try squatting or putting your one foot up on the toilet. Make sure that the cotton string is hanging down from the tampon when you insert it. Use your finger to locate the entrance to the vagina, which is just below your **urethra** (where your pee comes out).

The first few times you try to insert a tampon, you might want to use a dab of water-based lubricating jelly (such as KY jelly) on the tip of the tampon to help with insertion (never use oil-based lubricants such as Vaseline since they tend to hang around in the vagina attracting bacteria. The bacteria can potentially lead to infection, so it's best to use only water-based lubricants in the vagina). If you don't have any water-based lubricating jelly, ask your mom or pick some up at the drugstore in the feminine hygiene aisle. The lubricating jelly makes it a little easier to insert the tampon when you are learning and it can help if the vagina is dry and your flow is very light.

2. Hold the tampon with your thumb and middle finger. Locate your vaginal opening and place the tampon in the entrance to the vagina. Wiggle it around until you've got it in place and then slowly push it up into the vagina. The vaginal entrance usually tilts towards your lower back so you might have to play with the angle a bit before you get it right. When it is in far enough you'll feel a little resistance. This is because the tampon has hit the **cervix**, or the entrance to the uterus.

If you find it difficult to insert or push the tampon up into the vagina you might just be too nervous. Being nervous can make it difficult to relax the muscles in the vaginal entrance. Take a deep breath and slowly let the air out.

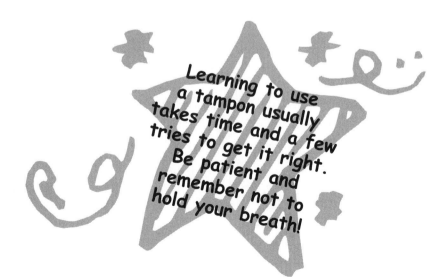

Learning to use a tampon usually takes time and a few tries to get it right. Be patient and remember not to hold your breath!

3. Once the applicator is half-way into the vagina, you can use your other hand to slowly push the tampon out of the applicator and into the vagina (remember to throw the applicator in the trashcan – don't try to flush it down the toilet). When the tampon is inserted correctly, you should feel no pain or discomfort. In fact, when a tampon is correctly inserted you should not be able to feel it at all. If you do feel it, it might not be in correctly.

Some girls like to use tampons without applicators. I was never a big fan of these because they can be really difficult to insert correctly. However, they are easier to carry with you, and you should know how to use one just in case you have an emergency and that's all a friend has to give you!

A tampon without an applicator is inserted the same way an applicator tampon is, but since there is no applicator to push it along, you use your finger to push it up into the vagina. Push it up as far as it will go until it meets resistance. Sometimes tampons without applicators can be difficult to insert if the vagina is dry and there isn't much flow. If this is the case, water-based lubricating jelly can be used.

4. Once a tampon is properly in place, the string will hang down outside of the vagina. You can push the string back up into the vaginal lips, where it will stay neatly tucked away (especially important when you're swimming or doing gymnastics – which reminds me of yet another story. One of the girls I interviewed told me about an experience she had in a gymnastics competition. After her balance beam event, she realized her tampon string had been hanging outside her leotard!) Tucking the tampon string away will ensure it won't hang where it's not supposed to. When you are ready to take the tampon out, you can just spread the vaginal lips, locate the string, and pull it out.

It's important that a tampon is never left inside the vagina for longer than eight hours because doing so can increase the risk of **toxic shock syndrome (TSS)**. Toxic shock syndrome is a bacterial infection that can develop when a tampon is left in place too long. Tampons provide a moist and warm place for bacteria to grow. While originally linked to tampon use, toxic shock can also be caused by other things such as surgery or illness.

How do you take out a tampon?

What goes up must come down, right? A tampon that is correctly inserted will not fall out by itself. To take it out, first position yourself over the toilet, just in case any menstrual fluid comes out while you're taking out the tampon. Gently pull the string and the tampon should slide out of the vagina. If you have minimal menstrual flow the tampon will be dry and hard to pull out. This is because the cotton is dry and the vaginal walls are not lubricated. Remember to be patient and breathe! Getting frustrated or nervous can make it harder to get the tampon out.

Sometimes you might have trouble finding the tampon string. It usually hangs out of the vaginal opening, but if the string was crooked in the applicator, it might not hang out. Don't panic! Just sweep your middle finger around the inside of your upper vagina and you'll find the string.

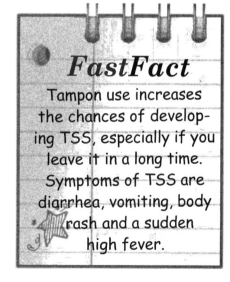

FastFact

Tampon use increases the chances of developing TSS, especially if you leave it in a long time. Symptoms of TSS are diarrhea, vomiting, body rash and a sudden high fever.

The tampon will never get lost inside of you because the vagina is only about four inches deep. If you squat over the toilet and bear down (like you are pooping), it might make it easier to feel the tampon in the vagina. With patience, you'll be able to easily pull it out.

If you pull and the string separates from the tampon, don't worry - you won't be making a trip to the emergency room! Wash your hands and using your middle finger, sweep the inside of the vagina as far up as you can reach. When you feel the tampon, gently nudge it out of the vagina.

Once a tampon is removed, always wrap it in toilet paper and place it in the trashcan. Don't flush it down the toilet, since this could lead to an embarrassing toilet overflow.

Do periods cause pimples?

Menstruation is controlled by changes in hormone levels. The rising and falling of these hormones may make pimples more likely during certain times of the month. However, periods don't cause pimples. Pimples are caused by blocked skin pores or oily skin and can be made worse by stress, eating the wrong foods, vitamin deficiencies, and many other things. If you do notice you get more pimples during your period, it's best to be careful about eating healthy foods (watch your sugar and salt intake) and make sure you keep your face washed. Exercise can also help increase blood flow and reduce pimples. The good news is that pimples associated with periods tend to be less of a problem as you get older.

Does every girl have cramps? How can I reduce them if I do?

Not all girls experience cramps when they menstruate, but those who do usually notice them during the first few days of their period. Cramps are caused by prostaglandins, which are natural chemicals in the body that cause the uterus to contract. Prostaglandins make the blood vessels to the uterus constrict so that the uterus gets less blood. When the uterus gets less blood, the inside layer breaks away, leading to menstrual flow. It's often easier to understand if you think about the job the uterus has to do. Cramps are muscle contractions designed to empty the uterus. They can vary from a dull and achy type of pain to sharp and intensely painful cramps.

Sometimes over-the-counter medications (those you can buy at the drugstore without a doctor's prescription) can help reduce cramps (such as Tylenol, Pamprin, or Midol). A hot bath or a warm heating pad can also help lessen the pain of cramps.

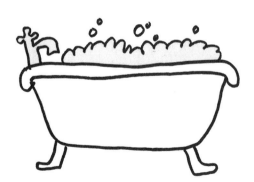

Regular exercise can also help. Exercise releases endorphins, which are natural painkillers produced by the body. These endorphins help reduce menstrual cramps. Exercise can also slow down the production of prostaglandins and help reduce mood swings and feelings of depression or anxiety, which are also common during menstruation.

Now you are an official period expert! I hope you feel more informed and confident about your period after learning the facts. However, there is one important question about periods that I didn't answer in these first two chapters. That is..."*why do periods happen?*" The answer to this question requires a little review of biology. In the next chapter we'll look at what actually goes on in your body to make a period happen.

The Science of Periods:
Fallopian Tubes, Breast Buds, and Hormones

The most complex question to answer is *"why do periods happen?"* To answer this question we'll need to start at the beginning. When you were born your body had all the parts necessary to one day make a baby. You had a **uterus**, **Fallopian tubes**, **ovaries**, and a **vagina** in your lower abdomen (called your **pelvis**). Your ovaries were stocked full of immature eggs, called **ova**. In fact, you were born with over 500,000 ova!

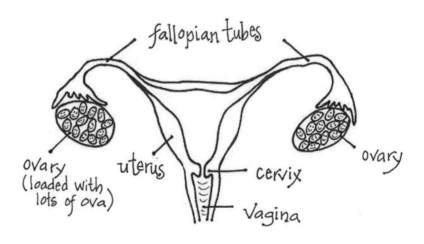

At birth and for many years afterwards, these ova just hang out in your ovaries until shortly after puberty begins. You will never make more ova – you are born with all you'll ever have (this is different than what boys experience; they begin to manufacture sperm during puberty, and they will make new sperm each and every day for their whole life). But girls never have to make more ova - we are complete when we are born!

Sometime between the ages of 8-12 years hormones in your body tell your ovaries to begin producing estrogen while you sleep. This is the beginning of puberty, and as it continues, the ovaries release estrogen into your circulatory system during the day and night. Increases in estrogen will have many effects on your body.

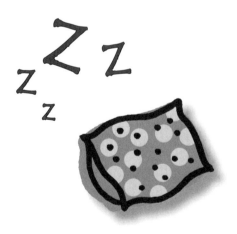

The changes you'll probably notice first will be in your breasts. Estrogen causes the nipples of the breasts to become very tender as the **breast buds** develop. Soon after this, **pubic hair** will begin to grow just above the vaginal opening and on the **labia majora**. You'll probably notice other body hair beginning to grow as well (such as under your arms or on your legs). Other important changes include increases in height, weight, a widening of the hips, skin changes (the skin usually softens), and an increase in perspiration. Typically, about 2 to 2 ½ years after your breast buds develop you'll experience your first period. The scientific name for your first period is **menarche**.

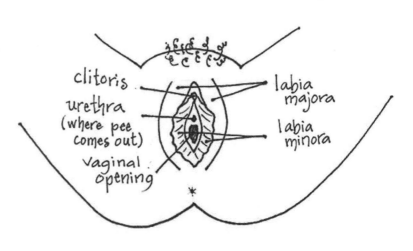

clitoris
urethra
(where pee
comes out)
vaginal
opening

labia
majora

labia
minora

what's what

About six months before your first period comes you might notice an increase in your **vaginal discharge**. There might be a white or yellowish discharge in your underwear. This discharge is very normal and it happens to all girls. There is no reason to worry about it unless it's itchy, painful, or has a strong odor (these symptoms might mean you have a vaginal infection). If you notice this make sure you tell your mom or another trusted adult. However, an increase in the amount of discharge just before your period is normal.

Typically, girls get their period anytime between the ages of 9-16 years old. Most girls get their periods around the age of 12 or 13 years old, but it's perfectly normal if it happens earlier or later. Menstruation represents a major stage of puberty in girls and it is one of the physical signs that a girl is becoming a woman.

It's a pretty cool thing to realize how much is going on in your body in order for you to get your first period. There are many different hormones involved and a complex interaction between these hormones, your brain, and your body. The hormones in your body interact with your reproductive organs, including the uterus, ovaries, and Fallopian tubes. It's easier to understand it if you think about a thermostat. A thermostat works by maintaining a certain temperature in your house. When the thermostat is set at 65° it will work to keep the room at this temperature. When the room gets colder, the thermostat will signal the furnace to produce more heat. When the room gets warmer than 65°, the thermostat will signal the furnace to turn off.

Your hormonal system works a lot like a thermostat. Your ovaries are responsive to hormone levels and when your body is ready, your hormonal system clicks into gear. Your **pituitary gland** produces FSH (follicle stimulating hormone) and LH (luteinizing hormone) which are chemical messengers (think of them like little mail-ladies....they carry the message from one place to the other). FSH and LH stimulate the ovaries to begin producing **estrogen**. Although both men and women have estrogen in their bodies, women have much more. Estrogen is responsible for many things in a woman's body, including the physical changes of puberty (breast development and changes in fat deposits) and the menstrual cycle. It is also responsible for the buildup of the uterine lining which will result in a period.

Once the ovaries have produced enough estrogen, chemical messengers in the brain tell the pituitary gland to stop the production of FSH and LH. Lowering levels of FSH and LH tell the ovaries to stop producing estrogen. Your menstrual cycle is an amazing system and one that we could never replicate, not even in your science class. (I dare you to ask your science teacher to try though!)

Shortly after your first period begins a few ova will begin to mature in your ovaries in preparation for **ovulation** (in fact, less than 500 of your 500,000 ova will actually be released in your lifetime – you are born with a gazillion more than you'll ever need). When ovulation finally happens, a tiny **ovum** will be released from one of your ovaries (sometimes it will come from the left ovary and sometimes from the right – you might be able to feel a little cramp or muscle twinge when the egg is released). The egg travels down one of the Fallopian tubes towards the uterus.

In the days before ovulation, hormones prepare the lining of your uterus (the **endometrium**) to build up and become thick and cushioned. If the egg were to become fertilized by a sperm (the male reproductive cell) it would implant into the soft, cushioned endometrial lining of the uterus. When this happens a woman becomes pregnant and usually stops menstruating.

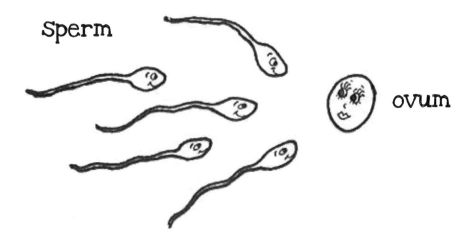

Sperm

ovum

However, during most of your menstrual cycles the egg will not become fertilized and you will have a period. The endometrial lining will be released through the vagina. In an average woman this cycle happens every month and continues until **menopause**, when a woman no longer releases ova from the ovaries and menstruation stops (this usually doesn't happen until a woman is 50-years old or so).

You might wonder why the uterine lining doesn't stay thick every day instead of going through such a complicated series of changes. This is an excellent question! The fluctuating hormone levels and the endometrial changes in the uterine lining each month help your body get ready to support a pregnancy one day.

So, now we've answered the question "*why do periods happen?*" It all seems so complicated, but in actuality it's really pretty simple. Your body knows what it's supposed do and no one has to tell it! Think about it this way - we have a really neat design that allows us to do something a boy can never do…….make and grow a baby! We are so lucky (I promise you'll think this is cool one day).

Now.....while all this biology stuff is going on in your body sometimes you might feel a little more emotional or sensitive to what's going on around you. In the next chapter, I'll tell you about emotional changes and what to expect during your menstrual cycle.

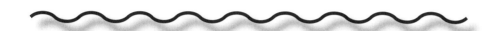

Chapter 4

The Emotions of Periods:
Happy, Sad, Tearful, and Joyful

Have you ever felt so happy and then, for no reason, just felt like crying? Emotional reactions like these are completely normal – especially when you're getting ready for your period. Some girls feel changes in their moods just before their period comes or during their period. It's common to feel like no one understands you anymore. You might feel irritated, angry, depressed, or just blue. You might cry more than usual

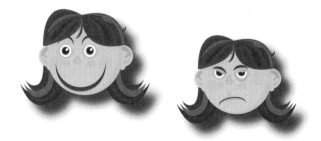

but not understand why. Some girls say they feel more anxious, aggressive, or even totally exhausted just before a period comes. If you feel any of these emotions, it's important to understand that you're not alone.

These emotional reactions are due, in part, to the hormonal changes associated with menstruation and are part of **premenstrual syndrome** (or PMS for short). Changing hormonal levels can affect the way you feel physically, emotionally, and mentally. One minute you feel confident and happy, and the next minute you're down in the dumps.

Medical experts have found more than 150 symptoms associated with premenstrual syndrome! It is estimated that over 85% of girls and women experience at least one of these symptoms as part of their monthly cycle. Common symptoms include trouble concentrating, remembering or focusing, increased tension, irritability, crying spells, mood swings, depression, low energy, and sleeping problems. Some girls say they have certain food cravings or find themselves eating more food than they'd like during this time. These symptoms vary from one woman to another and even from month to month in the same woman!

In addition to these emotional symptoms, some girls report feeling physical symptoms such as breast swelling and tenderness, backaches, headaches, and an increase in bloating, gas, constipation, and/or diarrhea. If you experience any of these physical or emotional symptoms, you might try keeping track of them on a calendar so you can see if there are any patterns in your symptoms. A "symptom diary" can help you understand more about the changes going on in your body.

It's important to point out that not all girls feel more emotional before their period. In fact, some girls have very few emotional and/or physical reactions to their menstrual period. The majority of girls who do say they have emotional or physical changes during their monthly cycles report these symptoms as mild. However, between 3-8% of women have a more severe form of PMS and they experience much more intense emotional and physical symptoms.

There are many things you can do to help reduce the emotional and physical changes associated with your menstrual cycle. Talk to your doctor or medical provider about taking a multivitamin with folic acid and calcium since this has been found to help ease some of these symptoms. Taking care of yourself and getting adequate exercise can help. Regular exercise can make you feel better both physically and emotionally. Even a short walk around the block or some jumping jacks can give you an extra boost of energy during this time.

It's also important to make sure you are eating healthy foods, including fruits, vegetables, and whole grains. Avoid eating lots of sugary or salty foods and limit the amount of caffeine you have. Caffeine, sugar, and salt can lead to water retention and bloating so it's best to drink lots of water when you're thirsty.

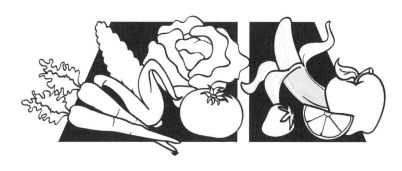

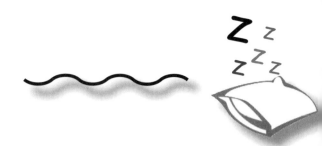

You'll also want to make sure you're getting at least eight hours of sleep a night. Less than this can make it more difficult for you to fight off feelings of sadness and anxiety. Over-the-counter pain relievers, such as Tylenol, can help reduce backaches, headaches, and breast tenderness. Not all of these work for everyone, so it's important to try some things out to see what works best for you.

It's common to have mixed feelings about getting your period. One of the best ways to deal with all of the physical and emotional changes is to learn why they happen AND ways to help make yourself feel better. What is something you like to do that makes you feel good? Is it grabbing a good book and finding a quiet space? Going on a bike ride or hike on a beautiful day? Talking with a friend? Listening to music? Finding what makes you feel good can help reduce the symptoms associated with your period.

In Their Own Words:
Mom, Menstruation, and Memories

In my conversations with girls, I've heard funny stories and I've heard scary stories. I've talked to girls who wished they would have known more about what to expect and others who didn't want to know anything. Some girls felt totally prepared, while others felt they were in the dark. When I first started this project I worried that girls might not feel comfortable talking to me about their periods. However, I realized pretty quickly that I was wrong. Not only did girls want to talk and tell their stories.....they had lots to say!

In this chapter, I'd like to share with you some of my conversations with hundreds of girls all over the country. I'll tell you who they talked to about periods, what they learned, where they were when they got their first period, and what they experienced. I hope that in reading this you'll understand the wide range in experiences, thoughts, emotions, and reactions.

Most girls talk to their Mom about menstruation before their first period.

While it's true that not all moms do it the same way, most girls do talk to their mom about Aunt Flo's visit BEFORE she arrives. Some moms make a point of sitting down with their daughters before the first period - they might give their daughter a book (hopefully this one!) or try to explain what to expect. Other moms wait until their daughters start menstruating to talk about it. Still other moms say nothing and expect their daughters to figure it out on their own.

Moms who say nothing often have moms who never talked to them about this important stuff. Since their moms never talked to them they think they don't have to talk to their daughters either. If this is your mom, remember that she might need a little help breaking the ice. Ask her questions! You might just find that she really wants to talk but didn't know how to start the conversation.

When I asked girls about these conversations with their mom, this is what they had to say:

"My mom told me that getting my period was perfectly normal and that all girls/women go through it. She explained it was a sign of getting older and maturing."

My mom told me that a period was an important step into womanhood and it was seen as a gift. She congratulated me when I first got my period and we had a small celebration. She also explained what I had to do when I got my period. Overall, it was really positive.

When I got my first period, I called my mom into the bathroom and she gave me a pad without saying a word. I remember looking at the back of the pad package to learn how to apply the pad. I had forgotten to take off the piece of paper that was on the back of the pad and I put the whole thing in my underwear. My friends were the ones who told me that I was supposed to peel off the paper so that the pad could stick to my underwear.

"My mom never said anything to me until after I got my first period. She just told me what was happening biologically."

" My mom never really explained it to me very much, but when I got my first period she bought me a book to explain everything. **"**

Few girls talk to their Dad about menstruation before their first period.

Talking to dad was a different story! In fact, I found that only 3% of girls had a conversation with dad about periods before they had their first period. Mom was clearly the one they talked to. Moms and daughters often have an easier time talking about these issues - but sometimes this makes dad feel a bit left out. Dads are definitely interested and many want to talk.

I know lots of dads who do an awesome job talk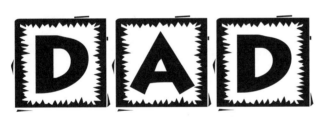ing to their daughters about growing up and and their first period. You might think your dad doesn't care or you might be too embarrassed to talk to him but the truth is that he might be respecting your privacy and is waiting for YOU to bring it up!

Many girls learn about menstruation in health class at school.

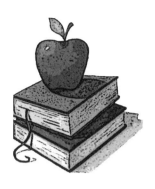

Although it's true that many girls learn something about puberty and body development in their health class at school, these classes often do very little to prepare a girl for her first period. In fact, the majority of girls I talked to told me that they wished they had learned more about what to expect during a first period in their health class. Remember that the school's job is to provide you with information about growing up -it's up to you to ask questions and fill in the blanks. Ask your mom, dad, teachers, or other trusted adults for more information!

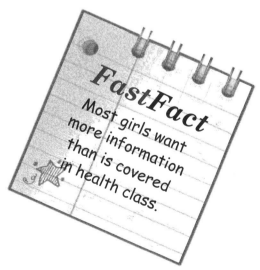

FastFact
Most girls want more information than is covered in health class.

The majority of girls worry about getting their first period.

Change is never easy but it's especially difficult when you feel unprepared for what to expect. The majority of girls I talked to told me that they were worried about what would happen when they got their first period. It's very common to feel worried or apprehensive about getting your period. Reading and learning can help you feel more confident and comfortable I hope you'll feel this way after reading this book.

Most girls are not expecting their first period when it comes.

Many girls told me that even though they were expecting their period to begin at some point, they were caught off-guard when it finally did arrive. Some were on their way to a sporting event, sleep over, or school. Below are some of their experiences:

> I was playing little league and I had two games in a row. I got it right before the second game. My mother took me to go get some pads and then I went and played the next game.

> I was in gym class when I got my first period. It was weird because I didn't know what was in my underwear. It didn't look like blood - at least not the color I was accustomed to seeing. It was brown and I panicked and asked to go to the nurse. The nurse assured me that yes, it was my period, and no, I wasn't dying. After being reassured, I remember feeling excited. Periods were COOL. Girls who got their periods were COOL. I was a woman! I couldn't wait to tell everyone. It was awesome.

> I was at the movie theater with my mother and sisters. I remember going to the bathroom and being in shock, then calling for my mom.

> I was playing a soccer game. It was the best game I ever played, I scored three goals and then got my period right at the end of the game.

I was outside playing in the woods with my older brother. I was scared and embarrassed so I ran inside for most of the day. I tried to hide what happened from my family, but my mom found out the next day when she did laundry. She was really happy and gave me a necklace and told me I had just become a woman. Then I felt better about the whole experience.

My parents were away and I was staying with my grandparents. I had a very close relationship with my grandmother and she explained everything to me. My older sister also helped explain what was going on.

I had just started 8th grade. I went to the bathroom and saw a dark reddish spot in my underwear. At first I didn't realize what it was, but once I did, I ran to the nurse and got a pad. Then I continued on my day.

I remember it was April Fool's Day so my mom didn't believe me...then I showed her my underwear. I had already put on a pad because I knew how to do it.

I was scared when I went to the bathroom and there was blood. I didn't know what was happening.

I woke up one morning and noticed blood. I yelled to my mom, "I'm bleeding!" I went to school and my mom wrote a note for me to bring to the school nurse so she would be aware if I went to her and wanted to go home.

I was at my house alone when I got my first period. My sister came home and gave me a maxi pad. When I told my mom, her reaction was neutral.

I was at home sleeping when I woke up to go to the bathroom in the morning and saw blood on my panties. I went up to my mother who was sleeping and told her I was bleeding. She congratulated me. I cried because I really did not want a period since it meant that I had to wear pads. When I told my friends everyone was excited and congratulated me.

I was at home when I got my first period. I had to go to school that day. I was really worried about people knowing and I worried that it would be obvious. My first period was definitely accompanied by a lot of embarrassment. It was something I just wished would just go away.

I woke up with my first period one morning. I didn't really know what was going on so I changed my underwear and it happened again. My mom walked in and saw my underwear. She got all excited and announced it to my dad.

I woke up one morning during the summer and saw that I had blood in my underwear. I screamed for my mom and she told me that I had gotten my period. She gave me some pads and told me how to use them.

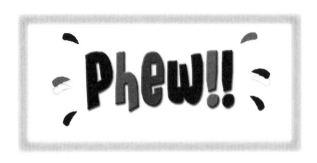

The majority of girls feel relieved or excited to get their first period.

While relief and excitement are common reactions to first periods, many girls feel a range of emotions when they start menstruating. Some feel apprehensive, worried, or even angry. A lot of your emotional reaction will be based on your expectations about your first period. You are much more likely to feel apprehensive if you don't feel prepared or if you are concerned that you won't be able to do certain things anymore (like play with your younger brother or sister!). When you are confident, informed, and prepared you are more likely to feel relieved and excited!

Many girls use "code" words to talk about their periods.

So I wasn't the only one! Menstruation code words are still common today. In fact, girls told me about lots of them. Some of my favorites were ...

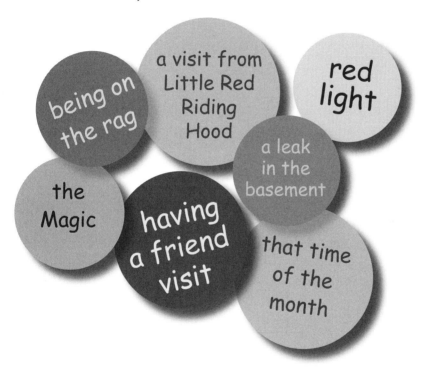

or my personal favorite,

the Red Sox are playing at home.

Code words like these can make it less embarrassing to talk about periods (especially around boys).

Most girls learn to use a tampon by themselves.

The majority of girls I talked to told me that they had to learn to use a tampon on their own. Some learned from friends or older sisters, but many reported feeling too uncomfortable to ask their mom for help. Moms might not want their daughters to use tampons or they might think a girl shouldn't use a tampon until she is older. They also might not know what to say or how to explain, so they just skip the whole thing. I think your mom is a great source of information and maybe you can start a conversation about tampons by asking her how old she was when she started using them. However, if you don't feel comfortable or if your mom doesn't say anything, don't forget to read page 30.

Many girls learn about using a pad from their moms.

While this is true, it's important to point out that not all moms offer the same type of directions. Some moms give detailed instructions, while others hand over the box of pads and point to the directions on the box.

Most girls have experienced an embarrassing moment with their period.

The majority of the girls I talked to could pinpoint at least one really embarrassing moment with their period. It happens to all of us! But the important thing to remember is that we get through these embarrassing moments just fine. The world doesn't stop and life goes on. Below are some of their experiences:

In 8th grade, I got my period in Spanish class and it bled through my underwear, my pants, and onto the seat. I didn't realize until I stood up to do a presentation in front of the class.

I was a sophomore in high school and I didn't know how to put a tampon in. I was at my friend's house and wanted to go in the hot tub but couldn't with a pad on. Having my friend tell me how to put in a tampon and demonstrate was embarrassing.

My period was really heavy and I didn't understand absorbency of different pads. So I had used a light pad on a very heavy day and blood got all over my chair in my sixth grade science class. The teacher was a guy and I was so embarrassed that when class ended I ran to my locker, tied a sweater around my waist and ran to the nurse. She sent me home early, which was nice.

I was not (and still am not) very good at keeping track of when I would get my period. One time I got my period in class while wearing WHITE pants. I had a HUGE blood stain because I hadn't noticed until far too late. I had to walk out in front of everyone to go to the nurse.

Probably the worst thing that ever happened early on with my period was one day when I got my period by surprise in class. A boy in my class asked what was all over my pants. I remember feeling extremely out of place because none of the other girls in my grade had their period yet. Once I realized that everyone had experiences like this I didn't feel so bad.

I was sitting in class in sixth grade and I felt my tampon leaking. I raised my hand to go to the bathroom and my teacher wouldn't let me go unless I answered his question in Italian class. So when I went to the bathroom, I leaked all over my beige overalls. I was really embarrassed, but luckily I had a sweatshirt to wrap around my waist.

I was always embarrassed that the sanitary pad's bulk would be visible to everyone and they would know that I had my period.

I remember being nervous that people would know I had my period. I kept a tin box of tampons in my locker. My girlfriends called it the "angel-box". They knew my locker combination, and could take one if they needed one.

The fact is almost every woman I've talked to about periods had at least one embarrassing moment to share. You might ask your mom, sister, girlfriend, or teacher about their most embarrassing moments associated with their periods. This might help jump start a conversation about periods (and you'll hear some pretty funny stories as well).

As you've read through these personal stories, I hope you've had a chance to reflect on the messages you have received about your period. Realizing what these messages were and learning all you can will empower you to sail right through these new experiences. Remember to take the time to get your questions answered and TALK to your mom and dad. If you find that your mom and dad are unable, or unwilling, to talk to you, find another trusted adult to talk to. You could talk to a relative, a friend's mom, teacher, school nurse, or even someone at your church or synagogue.

Getting your first period is really a time to celebrate. It's important to feel confident and prepared for your big day. There are lots of people around you who are willing and able to sit down and talk to you about periods. Don't let your fears or anxieties get in your way.

Finally....... don't ever forget that being a girl is awesome. You have so many wonderful opportunities waiting for you. Probably the most important thing you can do is sit back, relax, and learn to...

GO WITH THE "FLO"!

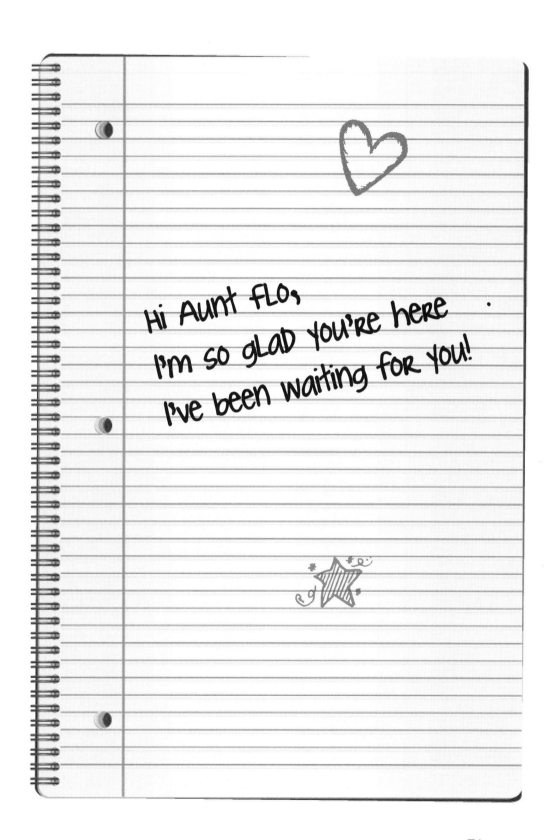

Hi Aunt Flo,
I'm so glad you're here
I've been waiting for you!

End Notes: Getting More Information

So, where can you go from here? Well, there are many people in your life that you could talk to and I'd really encourage you to do so. You might find that people are much more willing to talk than you think. Talk to your mom, dad, sisters, grandma, aunts, or other trusted adults. You can also talk to your friends, although keep in mind that sometimes friends don't know all the answers (even though they act like they do!).

Another great place to find information about puberty and menstruation is from books and Internet sources. Before checking out any Internet sources make sure you ask your parents for permission to go online.

Thanks for taking the time to read this book. I hope you leave with much more information than you started with and that you feel confident, prepared, and even a little bit excited. After all, it's not every day that you have something THIS special happen.

Glossary

Structure	Definition	Function
breast buds	The first swelling of the area around the nipple that indicates the beginning of breast development. Can be soft or firm to the touch.	Changes in breasts help prepare for potential breastfeeding later in life.
cervix (SUR · viks)	The doughnut-shaped lower part of the uterus that sits at the top of the vagina.	The shape of the cervix is controlled by hormones and can allow uterine discharge to pass.
cramps	Painful spasms of the uterine muscles, which can cause abdominal, back, and leg pain.	Helps dislodge the endometrial layer of the uterus - leading to menstrual flow.
endometrium (en · doh · MEE · tree · uhm)	The innermost, mucous membrane lining of the uterus.	Layer of tissue is responsive to hormonal changes and can support a pregnancy later in life.
estrogen (ES · truh · jun · n)	Important female sex hormone.	Responsible for many things including menstruation and the changes associated with puberty.
Fallopian tubes (fal ·OH · pee · in)	Two long slender tubes that extend from the ovaries to the uterus (named after Gabriele Falloppio who discovered the tubes in the 16th century).	Transport ova from the ovary to the uterus.
irregular cycle	Menstrual cycles that do not come on a regular schedule.	

Structure	Definition	Function
labia majora (LEY · bee · uh muh · JAWR · uh)	Two large folds of skin that lie outside the vaginal opening.	Protects the vaginal opening and contains sweat and oil glands to lubricate the vaginal opening.
menarche (MEN ·ark ; also pronounced Men · NAHR · kee)	The first period which marks the beginning of menstruation.	Begins the monthly menstruation cycle.
menopause (MEN · uh · pawz)	The end of menstrual cycling.	Hormonal changes in the body end ovulation, which in turn end the monthly cycle.
menstrual flow (MEN · stroo · uhl)	The blood and fluid that comes out of the vagina during a menstrual period.	To remove endometrial lining from the uterus.
menstruation (men · stroo · EY · shuhn; also pronounced mens · STREY · shuhn)	The scientific name for the monthly shedding of the uterine lining.	Prepares the body for another monthly cycle of ovulation.
ova (OH · vuh)	Female reproductive cells; also called eggs (single egg is referred to as an ovum)	Joins with male reproductive cell (sperm) to create a baby
ovaries (OH · vuh · rees)	Female reproductive organs that produce ova (eggs) and the hormone estrogen.	Produces and stores ova and manufactures the female hormone estrogen.
ovulation (OV · yuh · ley · shun)	The phase of the menstrual cycle in which an ovum is released.	Important role in pregnancy.
ovum (OH · vuhm)	The female reproductive cell; the egg (more than one is called ova).	Important role in pregnancy.
pelvis (PEL · vis)	The lower part of the abdomen, located between the hip bones.	Supports the pelvic organs.

Structure	Definition	Function
period	The slang term for the monthly bleeding that the majority of women experience.	Prepares the body for monthly cycles of ovulation.
pituitary gland (pi·TOO·i·ter·ee)	An important endocrine gland that lies at the base of the skull and secretes hormones into the bloodstream.	Regulates many bodily functions including growth, blood pressure and metabolism.
pre menstrual syndrome (pre·MEN·stroo·ul SIN·drome)	A range of physical and emotional symptoms that some women experience prior to their monthly periods.	n/a
pubic hair (PYOO·bik)	Hair growth in the pubic area.	Helps cushion and protect the female genitals.
toxic shock syndrome (TSS) (TOK·sik·shock SIN·drome)	A bacteria-caused illness that can lead to high fever, vomiting, diarrhea, sore throat, and can be fatal if left untreated.	n/a
urethra (you·REE·thruh)	Tube that extends from the urinary bladder to the outside of the body.	Allows urine to exit the body.
uterus (YOO·tuh·uhs)	The hollow muscular organ that is the site of menstruation.	Holds the developing fetus during pregnancy and provides muscular contractions during menstruation and labor.
vagina (vuh·JAHY·nuh)	A thin-walled muscular tube that leads from the uterus to the outside of the body.	Used as a passageway for menstrual fluid and a newborn baby.
vaginal discharge (VAJ·uh·nl dis·CHARGE)	A release of fluid from the vagina.	Removes unnecessary fluids from uterus and vaginal canal.

Put an X on the day your period begins and an X on the day it ends.
Count the days in between to see how often your period will come.

January

1	2	3	4	5	6
7	8	9	10	11	12
13	14	15	16	17	18
19	20	21	22	23	24
25	26	27	28	29	30
31					

February

1	2	3	4	5	6
7	8	9	10	11	12
13	14	15	16	17	18
19	20	21	22	23	24
25	26	27	28	29	30
31					

March

1	2	3	4	5	6
7	8	9	10	11	12
13	14	15	16	17	18
19	20	21	22	23	24
25	26	27	28	29	30
31					

April

1	2	3	4	5	6
7	8	9	10	11	12
13	14	15	16	17	18
19	20	21	22	23	24
25	26	27	28	29	30
31					

May

1	2	3	4	5	6
7	8	9	10	11	12
13	14	15	16	17	18
19	20	21	22	23	24
25	26	27	28	29	30
31					

June

1	2	3	4	5	6
7	8	9	10	11	12
13	14	15	16	17	18
19	20	21	22	23	24
25	26	27	28	29	30
31					

July

1	2	3	4	5	6
7	8	9	10	11	12
13	14	15	16	17	18
19	20	21	22	23	24
25	26	27	28	29	30
31					

August

1	2	3	4	5	6
7	8	9	10	11	12
13	14	15	16	17	18
19	20	21	22	23	24
25	26	27	28	29	30
31					

September

1	2	3	4	5	6
7	8	9	10	11	12
13	14	15	16	17	18
19	20	21	22	23	24
25	26	27	28	29	30
31					

October

1	2	3	4	5	6
7	8	9	10	11	12
13	14	15	16	17	18
19	20	21	22	23	24
25	26	27	28	29	30
31					

November

1	2	3	4	5	6
7	8	9	10	11	12
13	14	15	16	17	18
19	20	21	22	23	24
25	26	27	28	29	30
31					

December

1	2	3	4	5	6
7	8	9	10	11	12
13	14	15	16	17	18
19	20	21	22	23	24
25	26	27	28	29	30
31					

January

1	2	3	4	5	6
7	8	9	10	11	12
13	14	15	16	17	18
19	20	21	22	23	24
25	26	27	28	29	30
31					

February

1	2	3	4	5	6
7	8	9	10	11	12
13	14	15	16	17	18
19	20	21	22	23	24
25	26	27	28	29	30
31					

March

1	2	3	4	5	6
7	8	9	10	11	12
13	14	15	16	17	18
19	20	21	22	23	24
25	26	27	28	29	30
31					

April

1	2	3	4	5	6
7	8	9	10	11	12
13	14	15	16	17	18
19	20	21	22	23	24
25	26	27	28	29	30
31					

May

1	2	3	4	5	6
7	8	9	10	11	12
13	14	15	16	17	18
19	20	21	22	23	24
25	26	27	28	29	30
31					

June

1	2	3	4	5	6
7	8	9	10	11	12
13	14	15	16	17	18
19	20	21	22	23	24
25	26	27	28	29	30
31					

July

1	2	3	4	5	6
7	8	9	10	11	12
13	14	15	16	17	18
19	20	21	22	23	24
25	26	27	28	29	30
31					

August

1	2	3	4	5	6
7	8	9	10	11	12
13	14	15	16	17	18
19	20	21	22	23	24
25	26	27	28	29	30
31					

September

1	2	3	4	5	6
7	8	9	10	11	12
13	14	15	16	17	18
19	20	21	22	23	24
25	26	27	28	29	30
31					

October

1	2	3	4	5	6
7	8	9	10	11	12
13	14	15	16	17	18
19	20	21	22	23	24
25	26	27	28	29	30
31					

November

1	2	3	4	5	6
7	8	9	10	11	12
13	14	15	16	17	18
19	20	21	22	23	24
25	26	27	28	29	30
31					

December

1	2	3	4	5	6
7	8	9	10	11	12
13	14	15	16	17	18
19	20	21	22	23	24
25	26	27	28	29	30
31					

Notes

Notes

Notes